Disclaimer

The information in this eBook reflects the opinions of the author and is not intended to replace medical or psychological advice, or any other professional advice. This EBook is not intended to diagnose or treat any psychological or medical conditions or disorders. If you are in need psychological or medical treatment, consult with a certified and licensed professional before determining whether the information in this book should be used.

Preface

Hair fall today has been a major problem for the people who face this problem in there teenage.

Hair fall can increase very fast unless if not cured correctly and timely. Let us read in this book How to control and cure hare fall.

This book has been published for the wellness of the people who are suffering this problem. Lets read.

Hair Fall Control – Cure at Home

Hair loss is common problem that everyone faces at one point. Read these quick tips & home remedies for effective hair fall treatment.

It is said that hair is your health barometer and if you're seeing more of it on your pillow or in the shower, there's no need to ring any alarm bells. Losing about 100 hairs on a daily basis is a common occurrence. It happens when you comb your hair or even when you just do nothing. But new ones grow and replace them.

Excessive hair loss is attributed to a number of reasons - genetics, illness, medications, or even a poor diet. It can be extremely disturbing and embarrassing and there are two approaches to hair loss prevention – medical intervention and diet.

When in doubt, see a dermatologist. He will be able to recommend a topical application or a pill. These can be quite effective but the drawback is that they work for only as long as they are used. Your hair will start falling when you quit.

Hair replacement is another option available to both men and women. Some of the common methods are hair grafts and scalp reduction. Hair grafting is an outpatient procedure done at the dermatologist's office. Several sessions are usually required to achieve a natural look.

Scalp reduction surgeries are just what they sound like. Skin which doesn't have hair is surgically removed so that it looks like one has a full head of hair. It can be performed in conjunction with hair grafting.

Hair Fall Treatment - Simple Home Remedies to Control Hair Fall Effectively:

The Do's:

Coconut milk is a great source of nutrients. Massage it on the scalp to reduce hair fall.

Aloe vera gel also works wonders. Massage the scalp with aloe gel, leave in for a few hours and then wash with lukewarm water. Aloe gel, coconut milk and wheat germ oil make a great hair conditioning treatment to help fight hair fall.

The hot oil hair massage is an indulgence that is so typically Indian that many of us don't realise how it helps. Massages help stimulate blood flow to the scalp. Choose coconut, olive, mustard or almond oil for best results. Getting a head massage has two advantages – stimulating hair follicles and also making you feel relaxed.

Indian herbs like neem and amla steeped in massage oil are great hair fall treatment options.

In case of really severe hair fall, use hair packs made with eggs or yogurt to soothe the scalp and nourish hair. Of course, hair spas salons are equally effective.

Be mindful of what you eat – bad food habits coupled with stress will result in hair loss. Eat a balanced diet.

The Dont's:

Rubbing wet hair vigorously will lead to breakage. Avoid brushing wet hair for the same reason.

Don't tie your hair tightly all the time as it puts pressure on the roots and causes hair to fall.

Heat in any form is bad for hair. Hot water, hair dryers and hair styling tools dry out the hair. Limit the usage. fight-hair-fall

Get a trim regularly to keep split ends at bay.

Try not to use too many hair products as residue can build up. Rinse shampoo well to make sure hair follicles are not clogged.

Make sure to follow product instructions carefully. If you use too much of a product, it could lead to more hair fall.

To solve your problem of hair loss, try some of these natural remedies. Also, following a proper diet will keep your hair healthy & help reduce hair fall. So, eat plenty of green vegetables and fresh fruits as much as possible. Rad how you can control hair fall with these 7 Yoga asanas.

Read more Beauty tips here.

Home remedies to control hair fall, boost the hair regrowth

Fenugreek for hair loss

One of the most effective home remedies to control hair loss is using fenugreek / methi. Seeds of fenugreek are rich in hormone antecedents that help in hair growth and repairs hair follicles. These seeds also contain nicotinic acid and proteins that strengthen the hair shafts and boosts hair growth.

So, now as you know, how much fenugreek seed can help to control hair fall and boost hair growth you must be anxious to know how to use them for hairs. Soak the fenugreek seeds in water overnight and grind it in the next morning to make a fine paste. Apply this fenugreek seed paste to the scalp and hairs and let it set for 30 minutes to one hour, covering your hairs with a shower cap so that it does not get dry. Rinse off with plenty of water, no need of using a cleanser or shampoo. Follow this process of treatment at least twice a week for a month to see effective results.

Aloe Vera for hair loss

Nowadays, excessive hair loss has become very common due to heavy pollution in the environment. You can use Aloe Vera as another effective home remedy for hair loss and quick hair growth. Usage of Aloe Vera can effectively reduce scalp problems like, flaking and itching. The mildly alkaline property of Aloe Vera helps in restoring the natural pH level of the scalp which promotes hair growth. Aloe Vera gel can be effective even for fighting dandruff. Take an Aloe Vera leaf, collect the pulp and apply it to the scalp and hairs. Leave it on for 45 minutes to an hour and wash off the hair with plenty of normal water. Follow this treatment for 3 – 4 times a week for better results.

Aloe vera for hair

Onion for fighting hair loss

If you are suffering from heavy hair loss, here is the most effective home remedy for controlling hair loss and boosting hair growth. The onion in your kitchen can actually do wonders for your hairs.The high sulfur content of onions capable to improve blood circulation to the hair follicles. Onion juice also enjoys anti -bacterial properties that can kill the germs and parasites. Prepare fresh onion juice by grinding an onion and squeezing out the juice. Apply it on to the scalp and leave it on for half an hour. Finally, wash off with a mild cleanser and plenty of water.

Onion juice for hair fall control

Hot oil massage to reduce hair fall

Lack of nutrition to the hairs is often a cause of excessive hair fall and hence hot oil massage can be very effective to control hair loss. Massage the scalp daily at least for few minutes with lukewarm oil. You can use any oil that is rich in Vitamin E. Coconut oil, almond oil, mustard oil, olive oil and jojoba oil are the best options at your hand. If you are experiencing hair loss due to dandruff, jojoba oil can be particularly effective.You can also opt for a mixture of all the oils to get the best results. Heat the oil lightly in an iron or steel container and massage your scalp and hairs with the oil. To get complete benefits of hot oil massage it is best if you can leave the oil on your hairs overnight and then wash off in the morning, otherwise shampoo the hair after 1 hour.

Sour curd as a hair fall solution

Curd is one of the most effective home remedies for hair loss. It can also help to get soft, smooth and shiny hairs.You can either apply the sour curd directly onto your scalp and hairs or mix 2 tablespoon of curd with 1 tablespoon of honey and apply the mixture to get the best effects.Leave the mask on for 30 minutes and then wash off with plenty of water.

Indian gooseberry to reduce hair fall

Do you know tho how to use Indian gooseberry / amla for controlling hair fall and boosting natural hair growth? Vitamin C deficiency can trigger hair loss and Amla is rich in vitamin C. Gooseberry can help to maintain a healthy scalp and it also promotes hair growth. Take a few Indian gooseberries, discard the seeds and grind the flesh to make a pulp. Mix this pulp with a few drops of lemon juice and massage your scalp with this mixture. You can also use the pulp directly without adding the lemon juice. Keep this on for an hour and wash off with plenty of water.

Stop hair loss due to dandruff

Licorice roots to stop hair fall

Are you looking for best herbal remedy to stop hair fall? Licorice is a herb that can be very helpful in preventing the hair loss and hair damage. Licorice helps in getting rid of scalp irritations and soothes the scalp. If dandruff is a cause of hair loss this remedy can be actually helpful.Soak few strands of licorice roots in milk overnight. In the morning grind the mixture to make a paste and apply this paste to the bald patches before going to the bed. Leave it overnight and shampoo in the morning.

Hibiscus leaves or flowers

Well, this is the best ayurvedic home remedy for hair loss. Hibiscus flowers and leaves can be very helpful in preventing hair loss and to promote hair growth. Hibiscus flowers are used as an effective cure for split ends and dandruff as well. Heat 12-15 hibiscus flowers in 2 tablespoons of coconut oil. Strain the solution and collect the oil. Apply this concoction to the scalp and hairs, leave overnight and wash in the morning. To use the hibiscus leaves, grind them into fine paste and apply the paste to the scalp and hairs. Leave it on for 30 minutes to 1 hour. Rinse off with plenty of water. This controls the hair loss automatically and promotes hair growth.

Hibiscus leaves for strong and long hair

Beetroot juice to stop hair fall

This is the finest kitchen remedy to stop hair loss and promotes hair regrowth. Beetroot is rich in phosphorous, calcium, protein, potassium, carbohydrates, vitamin B and C. These are very essential nutrients for hair growth. Drink beetroot juice daily or include it in your regular diet for fast and healthy hair growth. Alternatively you can also use beetroot leaves to your scalp and hairs. Boil the beetroot leaves in water and make a paste. Apply this thick paste to scalp and leave it on for 30 minutes. Rinse off with water. Follow this procedure at least twice in a week for better hair growth and quick results.

Coconut milk for hair regrowth

Coconut milk consists of fats and proteins. It promotes hair regrowth and controls hair loss. For quick results apply the coconut milk to the scalp and hairs. Grate the coconut and grind it in a mixer. You can extract the milk from this paste and apply the milk directly to the scalp and hair ends. Leave it on for 30 minutes to 1 hour and shampoo the hair afterwards. It will stops hair thinning and promotes hair regrowth.

Tea decoction for controlling hair fall

Make use of tea decoction for preventing hair fall. Tea is rich in tannic acid which can be helpful to control any scalp infection and to promote hair growth.Prepare a strong tea decoction by boiling 3 spoons of tea leaves in one cup of water and strain the liquid. Squeeze one lemon into the decoction. Mix it well and rinse your hair with this mixture after shampoo. Then wash off with fresh water. Don't use shampoo after using the tea rinse. This is very effective home remedy for hair loss.

Shana Seeds for boosting hair growth

Did you ever heard of stopping hair loss with shana seeds and it is also possible to make an ayurvedic solution for hair regrowth. This is a well- known Ayurvedic treatment that effectively prevents hair loss and promotes hair growth. Take 2 tablespoons of shana seeds powder and mix it with 1 tablespoon of coconut oil to make a paste. Now apply this paste to the scalp and the hairs. Concentrate on the hair roots. You can actually rub in the mixture onto your scalp and hairs as well. Wash off with a cleanser after 15 minutes.

Spinach and lettuce juice to stop hair fall

Here is the best way to stop hair loss. The goodness of Spinach and Lettuce are well-known to all. These green veggies are rich in vitamins and minerals. They are also high in Iron and Biotin content, both of which are vital for the health of hairs and hair growth. To get the goodness of Spinach and Lettuce you can include these vegetables directly into your daily diet. It is best suggested to eat them half- cocked or boiled to get the best effects. You can also make a smoothie with spinach and lettuce and drink it twice a day to ensure that your hairs are healthy.

Prevent hair loss due to pregnancy

Reduce hair fall with Egg white

Did you ever wonder how to reduce hair fall with eggs? Egg white is rich in protein and vitamins. It can nourish the hairs in the best way, promoting smooth & shiny hair. If you want long and strong hair, you must follow this tip. Just break some eggs, remember not to use the yolk. Collect only the egg white and apply it as a mask to the scalp and hairs. This treatment is very effective to control hair fall in case the hair fall is triggered due to lack of nourishment and dryness of the hairs. Wash it off with a cleanser after 30 minutes to 1 hour. It will make the hairs stronger and healthier. Repeat this treatment at least once in a week to reduce hair fall and boost hair growth.

Apple cider vinegar to reduce hair fall

Apple cider vinegar can be effective to control hair fall and it gives soft and manageable hairs. Mix one part of apple cider vinegar in one part of water. Take this mixture in a spray bottle and spray onto your scalp and hairs. Massage gently and leave on for 5 minutes before washing off with a mild cleanser.If you do not like the smell of ACV, just mix a little amount of your regular oil to the vinegar and use it. For better results make use of this treatment at least twice a week.

Juice of potato for controlling hair fall

Lack of vitamins and minerals can cause dry and brittle hairs which can trigger hair fall. Potato can be a good remedy to control hair fall in this case. Potato is rich in Vitamin B6, Vitamin C, manganese, phosphorus, copper and niacin which can be helpful for boosting hair growth. Crush some cleaned potato and squeeze out the juice. Now apply this fresh juice directly onto your scalp and hairs. Leave on for 30 minutes to an hour but do not let the pack get dry. Wash off with plenty of water.

Grape seed oil controls hair loss

Grape seed oil is an effective natural hair conditioner and moisturizer. It can address hair issues like hair loss, dandruff and weakened hair. You can use grapeseed oil as a regular hair care product to get healthy hairs. Grape seed oil contains anti-oxidants that might be effective to control DHT production at the hair roots, which happens to be one of the main reasons of hair fall. Simply massage your scalp and hairs regularly at night with this oil, let it seep in overnight and wash off with a cleanser in the morning.

Dandruff home remedies
Safflower oil for hair fall

For preventing hair loss and baldness safflower oil can be used. This oil is rich in monounsaturated and polyunsaturated fatty acids which are vital for healthy hairs. You can find two varieties of safflower oils in the market, both of which can be used for hair care. Safflower oil is helpful for permed, colored and dry hair. Use safflower oil for massaging the scalp. Leave it on overnight and rinse in the next morning. Use it every alternate day to get healthy hair.

Add Saw Palmetto supplement to your diet

A recent publication in a world renowned Journal mentioned that alternative and complementary medicine like saw palmetto (Serenoarepens) may increase hair regrowth in men. In the study, better hair growth was observed in men who took 400 mg palmetto in addition to 100 mg of beta-sitosterol (from saw palmetto) regularly. Historically, palmetto continues to be used by herbalists for curing thinning hair in both men and women.

Under-active thyroid gland (hypothyroidism) can cause hair thinning

Add vegetables like kelp, nori, dulse, kombu and wakame in your daily diet. These veggies are rich in iodine and can be helpful to ensure the right functioning of the thyroid gland. You also can take 100 mg or 1 mL of the herb bladderwrack (Focus vesiculosus) regularly for better thyroid functionality. If you think that you are suffering from an under-active thyroid gland visit a medical care professional.

Get enough fatty acids

Including essential fatty acids in your regular diet can be helpful to stop hair fall, promoting hair growth, naturally. Walnuts, nuts, flax seeds, almonds, fish and avocado are common natural sources of healthy fatty acids. So include these nuts and fruits along with fish in your daily diet. You can simply munch on walnuts and almonds. Use flax seeds in any of your diet; just ensure to chew them well. Fishes like Salmon and Tuna are the richest animal source of fatty acids.

Prevent hair loss during travel

Add biotin to your diet

Biotin has been found to be a very important component for the health of hair. Deficiency of biotin can cause hair fall and hair thinning.So, if you are suffering from hair fall, include foods that are rich source of biotin in your regular diet. Meat, seafood, soy beans, eggs, dairy products, nuts, green vegetables like cabbage, kale, broccoli and cauliflower and fruits like Avocado are rich source of biotin. So, include these foods in your diet and experience the change within weeks.

Increase keratin production with MSM

Methyl sulfonyl methane is great for producing keratin (a hair protein), which helps in strengthening hairs. A study found, all the people taking MSM experienced reduced hair fall combined with increased hair growth in only six months. Milk, tomatoes and corn are naturally rich in MSM and they can stop hair fall and are also very effective to boost hair regrowth. So, include these foods in your regular diet.

Rejuvenate hair follicles with B-complex nutritional vitamins

Taking 100 mg of any B-complex supplement daily helps in hair growth. It includes biotin and vitamin B6 that reduces hair fall by increasing the blood circulation in scalp and rejuvenating the hair follicles.These food supplements are effective and sure shot solution of hair fall, but it is best if you consult your doctor before taking any such supplements.

How to increase hair volume naturally

Increase collagen production with vitamin C

Collagen makes an essential element of the hairs but as we age collagen starts to break down, leaving hairs more prone to breaking. The best way to boost collagen level in your hairs is to increase the amount of Vitamin C in your daily diet. Foods naturally loaded with vitamin C include; citrus fruits, strawberries and red pepper. Including 250 mg of Vitamin C in your daily diet can help to boost the collagen production.

Prevent the breakage with vitamin e antioxidant

Vitamin E helps in nourishing damaged hairs and also prevents breakage. It aids the body's capability to produce more keratin to stop hair breakage. Adding 400 IU of Vitamin E antioxidant in your daily diet is a good idea to grow long and lustrous locks.However, before you start with any supplement consult your doctor first.

Eat foods rich in iron

Iron is an essential element for hairs. If you are suffering from excessive hair fall, iron deficiency can be a common reason. Iron is essential for hair growth and is available in blackstrap molasses, leafy vegetables, leeks, cashews, dry fruits, figs and berries. Meat and poultry are also rich in iron content. So, include these iron rich foods in your diet in proper quantity to ensure that you are not suffering from anemia. You can also take an iron supplement after discussing with your doctor to get quick results.

Iron rich foods

Boost scalp blood circulation with rosemary oil

Rosemary oil has been traditionally used to increase blood circulation on the scalp. Add a few drops of rosemary oil to your coconut fat and massage your scalp regularly with this mixture. This massage will effectively stops hair fall.

Give hair a nutrient boost

It has been found that minerals like silica and zinc are also critical for hair growth. These elements contribute to keep the scalp and hairs healthy. These trace elements are needed in little amount in our body, but if there is a deficiency of these minerals, it can trigger hair fall. Beans, cucumber, mango, celery, pumpkin seeds, oysters and eggs are natural sources of these minerals, so include these foods in your regular diet. You can also take 500 mg of silica twice a day in addition to 30 mg of zinc after consulting with your doctor.

Boost blood circulation in scalp with rosemary oil

Rosemary oil has been traditionally used to increase blood circulation on the scalp.This essential oil not only stops hair fall but also boosts hair growth. However, never apply any essential oil directly to your scalp or hairs. Add a few drops of rosemary oil to carrier oil like, coconut or almond or olive oil and massage your scalp regularly with this mixture. This treatment can stop hair fall effectively.

Causes of hair fall

Stress

Stress is also a primary reason of hair fall. Three types of hair fall are associated with stress;these are, trichotillomania, alopecia areata and telogen effluvium. Though the hair fall caused due to stress is not permanent, you can control this by doing yoga or meditation or any physical exercises.

Best hair oils for hair growth

Infections or fungal diseases

Hair fall may also occur due to infections. Fungal infection like ringworm can be a major cause of hair fall. Ringworm starts as a pimple and slowly spreads resulting into bald patches. Some infections can be controlled naturally over time but you need to identify the problem and opt for the best remedy at the earliest to stop hair fall.

Heredity

Heredity is considered as a primary reason of baldness. If it is there in your genes, you can hardly do anything to stop it. However, the chance of androgenetic alopecia is much rare in women due to their genetic makeup but even women can experience hair thinning or small bald patches due to heredity.

Insufficiency of nutrients

If there is vitamin or mineral deficiency in your body, your hairs are surely going to take the heat.Protein is also vital to make the hairs strong and healthy. So, ensure to intake a proper balanced diet rich with protein, vitamins and minerals.

Aging

Aging can also be a cause of hair thinning in some cases. This generally occurs due to lack of nutrients and collagen in the body. However, it is not an obvious reason and you may not suffer from hair fall and balding even if you get old if it is not there in your genes.

PCOS (polycystic ovarian syndrome)

In many women, PCOS is a primary reason of excessive hair fall. PCOS can be caused due to many reasons, starting from obesity to unhealthy lifestyle and hormonal imbalance. It effects the menstrual cycle in women and can trigger extreme hair fall. You need medical assistance to cure this condition.

Best shampoos to prevent hair fall

Pregnancy

One can experience heavy hair fall during or after the pregnancy. It is generally triggered by the changes in the hormonal levels in the body of the mother during pregnancy. However, the hair lost due to pregnancy usually comes back after delivery.

Use of styling tools and chemicals

Many people use styling tools for straightening hairs. Use of chemical filled sprays for achieving a desired hairstyle is also quite common. Use of heat and chemicals destroys the hair texture and makes it prone to damage. Donning very tight hairstyles can also affect the hair roots causing hair fall.

Medications

Certain medications can cause severe hair loss. Medications used for treating infections or hormonal imbalances can trigger hair fall in some cases. Consult your doctor immediately in case you notice extreme hair fall after taking a particular medication.

Some recent studies have proven that drinking, smoking and sun exposure can also cause hair loss.

Here are the top 10 home remedies for hair loss.

1. Hair Oil Massage

The first step that you can take to reduce hair loss is to massage your scalp with appropriate hair oil. Proper hair and scalp massage will increase blood flow to the hair follicles, condition the scalp, and enhance the strength of your hair's roots. It will also promote relaxation and reduce feelings of stress.

You can use hair oils like coconut or almond oil, olive oil, castor oil, amla oil, or others. Add a few drops of rosemary essential oil to the base oil for better and faster results. Other types of oil that you can use are emu oil, argan oil, and wheat germ oil.

Massage any of the hair oils mentioned above onto your hair and scalp by applying light pressure with your fingertips.

Do this at least once a week.

2. Indian Gooseberry

For natural and fast hair growth, you can use Indian gooseberry, also known as amla. Indian gooseberry is rich in vitamin C, of which a deficiency in the body can cause hair loss.

The anti-inflammatory, antioxidant, antibacterial, and the exfoliating properties present in Indian gooseberry can help maintain a healthy scalp and promote hair growth.

hair loss home remedy using amla or indian gooseberry

Mix one tablespoon each of Indian gooseberry or amla pulp and lemon juice.

Massage your scalp with the mixture thoroughly. Cover your hair with a shower cap.

Leave it on overnight and shampoo your hair in the morning.

3. Fenugreek

Fenugreek, also known as methi, is highly effective in treating hair loss. Fenugreek seeds contain hormone antecedents that enhance hair growth and help rebuild hair follicles. They also contain proteins and nicotinic acid that stimulate hair growth.

Soak one cup of fenugreek seeds in water overnight.

In the morning, grind them to make a paste.

Apply the paste to your hair and cover with a shower cap. After about 40 minutes, rinse your hair.

Follow this remedy every morning for a month.

4. Onion Juice

Onion juice helps treat hair loss due to its high sulfur content, which helps improve blood circulation to the hair follicles, regenerate hair follicles and reduce inflammation.

The antibacterial properties in onion juice also help kill germs and parasites, and treat scalp infections that can cause hair loss.

In a 2002 study published in the Journal of Dermatology, almost 74 percent of the study participants who applied onion juice on the scalp experienced significant hair regrowth.

Extract the juice of one onion by grating it and then strain it. Apply the juice directly onto the scalp. Leave it on for about 30 minutes, and then wash it off. Finally, shampoo your hair.

Mix together three tablespoons of onion juice and two tablespoons of aloe vera gel. You can also add one tablespoon of olive oil. Apply this mixture onto your scalp and leave it on for at least 30 minutes before rinsing it off and shampooing your hair.

Repeat either of these remedies two or three times a week for several weeks.

5. Aloe Vera

Aloe vera contains enzymes that directly promote healthy hair growth. Also, its alkalizing properties can help bring the scalp and hair's pH to a more desirable level, which can greatly promote hair growth.

Regular use can also relieve scalp itching, reduce scalp redness and inflammation, add strength and luster to hair, and alleviate dandruff. Both aloe vera gel and juice will work.

Apply aloe vera gel or juice onto the scalp.

Leave it on for a few hours and then wash it off with lukewarm water.

Repeat the process three to four times a week.

You can also consume one tablespoon of aloe vera juice daily on an empty stomach to enjoy better hair growth.

6. Licorice Root

Licorice root is another herb that prevents hair loss and further damage to the hair. The mollifying properties of licorice roots open the pores, soothe the scalp and help get rid of irritations like dry flakes. This remedy is good for dandruff, hair loss and baldness.

Add one tablespoon of ground licorice root to one cup milk with a quarter teaspoon saffron. Mix it thoroughly.

Apply the paste on bald patches at bedtime and leave it on overnight.

In the morning, wash your hair.

Follow this remedy once or twice a week.

You can also take licorice internally in the form of licorice tea three times a day.

Top 10 Tips to control Hair loss, Hair fall: Natural & Herbal Remedies

July 10, 2012 Health

Hair is one of the important components in human life to enhance one's beauty and complexion. It is the wonderful gift of nature that requires extra care and nurture. However, due to faulty lifestyle, paradox dietary pattern, junk food culture, etc., hair loss and hair fall is common among the masses, especially with women.

About 50% women faced hair loss at some stages of her life. Hair loss in women is demoralizing, may affect marital life, job opportunities, social adjustment, etc.

How to Control and Prevent Hair Loss?

Some asanas of Yoga is quite beneficial in prevention of Hair loss and Hair fall. Yoga augment blood circulation into the head and scalp region thereby strengthen hair root internally. Asanas like Shirsasana and Sarvangasana enhances blood circulation to the head and scalp region thereby facilitate hair growth.

Massage your head region with coconut oil or Vitamin E oil prevent hair loss.

Massage your scalp with Camphor + Coconut oil strengthen the root hair and prevent hair loss.

Massage with the mix of honey and egg yolk is quite beneficial in the management of hair loss.

Slow massage of the scalp portion stimulate blood circulation and helps in re-grow of hair.

If you want shining hair, use the mix of Amla, Shikaki powder and curd. This mixture helps to clean the pores of the scalp and stimulate hair growth.

Everybody has lemon in their home, rinse your hair with lemon juice to prevent baldbess.

Baldness can be cured if you apply the mix of curd, lemon and mustard oil on your head portion. Leave it for 30 minutes and wash it after then.

For shining and glow hair, one should eat more and more protein enriched foods such as fish, yeast, soybean, eggs and beans.

Activities like Hair dyes, hairdryer, curling, coloring, braids, buns, ponytails, etc. should be avoided. Shampoo, Conditioners, Alcohol and Beverages should be discouraged.

20 Simple Home Remedies To Control Hair Fall

Oct 24, 2014 Green Yatra BlogNatural Home Remedies0

7-simple-home-remedies-for-hair-fall-2Hair fall or alopecia is very embarrassing and you tend to feel helpless and confused. You try to hide the bald patches on your head. You try many hair fall products to solve the problem but still search for natural remedies to solve your hair fall problem. Many factors like genetics, thyroid disorders and anemia, chemical treatments can cause hair fall. You don't have to wait till 50 for hair fall to start! Every time you leave the shower, you see the drain clogged with hair. Even when you comb your hair, you see strands of hair on the comb. This is really frightening! It makes you wonder what can be the possible reason behind hair fall.

If hair fall is persistent, it is always best to contact a dermatologist and get his advice. He will probably give medicines like Minoxidil, Finasteride and Dutasteride to stimulate hair growth. Hair fall might start from a section creating a bald patch; this is commonly called alopecia areata.

Causes of Hair Fall:

So what is the solution to hair fall? Do anti-hair fall products really help? The answer is just look within. Yes internal problems also triggers hair fall. So before knowing how to prevent hair fall, we should know the reason behind it!

a. Lack of Proper Nutrition:

Hair is made up of a protein called Keratin. For the hair to grow you need to have proteins and iron along with essential vitamins. Ninety Percent of the hair is always in a growing phase, it takes two to three years for the hair to grow and then it enters a resting phase of three months. After that hair sheds and new hair takes its place. So to allow the hair growth you need the right blend of protein and iron. A balanced diet will surely give you healthy hair.

b. Aging:

With age hair starts thinning, this happens because the body's capacity to absorb nutrients decrease.The hair needs 22 amino acids to grow. Due to lack of amino acids from the diet the hair appears thin.

However you can prevent the hair fall due to aging. You need to have soy beans, lean meat, dairy products, fish, eggs and nuts. You can also have fish oil tablets or supplements which is rich in Omega 3 Fatty Acids.

c. Hormonal Changes:

Hair fall or alopecia happens due to high or low hormone levels. Hormones regulate all the organs in the body. Estrogen, progesterone, testosterone are the active hormones in a woman's body. Female pattern of baldness occurs when the dihydrotestosterone (DHT) levels increase in the scalp.

The dihydrotestosterone (DHT) is a byproduct of testosterone and it is produced in the follicles where enzymes convert testosterone into DHT. Sometimes genes are responsible in converting testosterone into DHT readily leading to baldness. Also when levels of female hormones decrease the male hormones become active leading to hair fall.

Also progesterone that is secreted in the body during ovulation decreases during menopause. The body produces adrenal cortical steroid called androstenedione. This steroid has male hormonal qualities that cause hair fall.

d. Stress:

Hair fall is caused due to stress.There are three types of hair fall that are associated with stress. They are:

Telogen Effluvium– Stress pushes the hair follicles into arresting phase. After a few days you will noticehair fall.

Trichotillomania– This is an irrestible urge to pull out hair from the head and eyebrows. Hair pulling can be triggered by emotions like stress, tension, loneliness, boredom and frustration.

Alopecia Areata– This type of hair loss is triggered by severe stress. Stress weakens body's immune system and causes hair fall.

However, hair fall caused due to stress is not permanent and it can be controlled. Just practice meditation or yoga to de-stress. Taking deep breaths and drinking water helps.

e. Heredity:

Androgenetic alopecia is caused by genetic and environmental factors. If anyone in your family has suffered alopecia, there are high chances that you will lose hair too. In women androgenetic alopecia doesn't cause total baldness but there is visible hair thinning.

f. Prolonged Illness:

Chronic and deadly diseases like cancer, typhoid and jaundice can trigger hair loss. Cancer medicines and chemotherapy cause severe hair loss. Beautiful hair is a reflection of good health, so if there is any problem with your general health it reflects on your skin and hair.

h. Thyroid Disorders:

People suffering from Hypothyroid and Hyperthyroidism lose hair. It is a worst symptom of thyroid and it is easily visible. However, it can be treated by doing a proper evaluation by your doctor. You need to give the hormones some time to stabilize. Also try to analyze the type of hair loss you are having and talk to an endrinocologist about it.

i. Fungal Disease or Infections:

Some infection causing agents are responsible for hair fall. Ringworm, which is actually not a worm, is a fungal infection that causes alopecia. The condition is called 'tinea capitis,' ringworm is same as athlete's foot. The ringworm starts as a pimple and it slowly spreads causing a bald patch. The affected area is itchy, red, inflamed and it may ooze.

Never share towels, combs and clothes. You can get fungal infection if you're a regular at swimming clubs, common showers is the place you can probably get these fungal infections.

j. Pregnancy:

Giving birth is quite scary for most women, in addition if you are losing bunches of hair it adds to the depression. It happens after the baby is delivered and hormonal changes are the main reason.

k. Over Styling Hair:

We all love to straighten our hair and highlight the hair with some funky colours to look trendy.Other chemical treatments like perming and rebonding can destroy the hair texture. Also using straightening rods and curlers cause strain to the hair and leads to hair breakage and split ends. Also using tight rubber bands and hair accessories can cause hair fall. Never tie a high ponytail, keep it loose and simple, you will still look pretty.

l. Excessive Vitamin A Intake:

According to American Academy of Dermatology hair fall is caused due to overdosing on Vitamin A. One should have only 5,000 International Units of Vitamin A. However this hair fall is temporary and can be corrected by reducing the Vitamin A intake.

m. Vitamin B Deficiency:

This problem of hair fall can be corrected and is very common. You just need to correct your diet. Having fish, meat, starchy vegetables, nuts and avocado can solve your hair woes. You can snack on nuts to get good hair.

n. Autoimmune Disease, Lupus Cause Hair Fall:

Lupus cause 'scarring', this means the hair will not grow back. All you have to do is to change your hair style to camouflage the bald patches. Short is better for camouflaging the baldness.

o. Dramatic Weight Loss:

Hair fall can be caused due to physical trauma. Eating disorders like Bulimia and Anorexia cause hair fall. So eating right to reduce chances of deficiencies is very important if you want your hair to shine with a healthy glow.

p. Polycystic Ovarian Syndrome (PCOS):

This is another case of hormonal imbalance. Excess of androgens cause ovarian cysts and affects your menstrual cycle. Polycystic ovaries cause hormonal imbalance and this leads to hair fall.

All the causes sound very common, yet we cannot control hair fall.

20 Simple and Effective Home Remedies to Control Hair Fall:

Latest technology and hair fall products claim to reduce hair fall and most of them are effective. However it is always better to go for natural products than opting for chemicals that harm the hair.To curb hair fall, you need to include a few basic practices into your hair care routine along with the treatments that you adopt for better results. Here are some home remedies and tips for hair fall control you can try.

1. Coconut Milk:

7 simple home remedies to control hair fall

Coconut milk is among the richest sources of tissue-nourishing, plant derivatives. Grind the grated coconut and squeeze it to remove its milk. Massage coconut milk on the scalp to reduce hair fall.

2. Aloe Vera:

7 simple home remedies to control hair fall

Aloe Vera juice is very effective to stop hair loss. Pure aloe gel can be applied directly to the scalp. This is helpful for preventing hair loss due to irritated, dry or infected scalp. Aloe Vera balances the pH level of scalp. After massaging the head with aloe gel, wait for few hours and then wash the hair with lukewarm water. You should do this twice a week for best results.

You can also make your own anti hair fall shampoo. Mix aloe gel, wheat germ oil and coconut milk. Apply this on your scalp and wash off

Another remedy is to dissolve a small amount of sodium chloride in the aloe vera gel. Now apply this mix on the scalp. The sodium will penetrate into the deeper layers of your skin and reduce hair fall.

3. Oil Massage:

Oil Massage

Regular massaging the scalp for a few minutes every day with lukewarm oil will lead to stimulation of blood flow to the scalp. Coconut oil helps in controlling hail fall. Other recommended oils are: Jojoba oil, almond oil, mustard oil, lavender oil. Jojoba oil is especially good because it replaces the sebum in the scalp. It also helps to control dandruff.

4. Neem Treatment:

Neem is one of the most popular herbs in the country! It has many benefits, both health and beauty. And when it comes to beauty, it has some very effective hair benefits too. The astringent property of neem helps to keep lice and dandruff at bay.

How to use:

Boil neem leaves in water until the water level falls to half its initial quantity and then cool it.

Rinse out your hair with the mixture once a week.

5. Amla:

Boil dried amla in coconut oil till the oil turns black in color. Massage your scalp with this oil. This is an effective and very easy home remedy to check hair loss. There are also other ways where we can include amla in our hair care routine. Here are some methods to use amla effectively to control hair fall:

Use amla and shikakai powder than you can buy in ayurvedic stores. Mix them both and make a paste. Apply this to your hair. Leave it on for a few minutes and wash off after a few minutes. Caution: If you have dry hair, skip shikakai.

Mix powdered amla with lime juice. Apply this on your scalp and leave on for some time. Wash off.

Soak it overnight. Use the water in the morning to rinse off your hair post shampooing.

The most effective method to reduce hair fall is to drink amla and shikakai juice. Yes, it tastes terrible but if you skip the preference of the taste buds once a day, the results will definitely be worth it.

[Read: How To Prevent White Hair]

6. Curd:

Curd is an excellent remedy for improving the quality of the hair and prevents hair loss as well. It ios one of the best conditioners and can be used in various forms:

Mix curd with black pepper. Apply this on your hair. Wash off thoroughly when dry

Mix curd with honey and apply this on your hair. Applying curd with honey or lime juice moisturizes your hair.

It also makes your hair shiny. This natural hair mask is also effective against dandruff which can be a cause of hair loss.

7. Hair Fall Preventive Packs:

When hair fall is really severe, then a preventive hair pack is the way to go. Here are a few packs, you can try at home.

Pack 1: Aloe Vera mixed with herbal Amla, shikakai and neem powder gives lustrous hair.

Pack 2: Henna, egg whites and curd when used together stops hair fall.

Pack 3: Honey, olive oil, cinnamon mixed together make for a soothing yet effective hair growth pack.

Pack 4: Wash your hair with a paste made out of neem leaves. Follow it up with rinsing your hair with apple cedar vinegar. Neem acts against scalp oil build up and infection while apple cedar vinegar maintains the alkali balance of the scalp.

You can always go for a hair spa once in a while but natural treatment is always a best idea. Stick to homemade hair masks to reduce hair fall. Keep your hair naturally hydrated.

[Read: Egg For Hair Fall]

8. No Junk Please:

7 simple home remedies to control hair fall

Unhealthy lifestyle, eating junk and all these unhealthy habits leads to hair loss. Processed foods are not healthy and it can cause diseases which ultimately lead to a rise in high level of toxins in the body. To counter the toxins you need to drink plenty of water. At least drinking 8 glasses of water on a daily basis is a must and preferably on an empty stomach.Eat fresh home cooked food if you want great hair.

9. Be Gentle With Wet Hair:

Avoid rubbing your hair dry and also avoid combing wet hair. Your hair is more susceptible to breakage when wet and the result will be a clump in your brush and stray strands at your feet.

10. Massage Your Scalp Frequently:

This stimulates blood circulation in the scalp and it also promotes hair growth. You can go for a hot oil massage and turban therapy to control hair fall. Make sure the oil is not too hot otherwise it will cause more harm than good. Listed below are some more ways of massaging the scalp:

Mix coconut oil, lime water and lime juice. Now apply this mix to get rid of hair fall

Hair massage can also be done with tree tea, olive oil, lavender oil, sesame oil or almond oil. All these oils are known to be good for preventing hair fall.

Massage the scalp with fresh coriander juice.

Boil 250 grams of henna leaves in mustard oil till only 60 grams of it is left. Store this and massage your hair with it.

Boil methi or fenugreek seeds in coconut or mustard oil. Regularly massage your hair using this preparation

Massaging scalp with coconut milk strengthens the hair. Grind coconut and strain all the liquid and you have natural coconut milk.

11. Minimize Pressure:

Don't always opt for styles that require you to tie your hair up tight. As sleek and fashionable as this may look, it puts a great deal of pressure on the hair which adds to the breakage and hair fall.

12. Avoid Excessive Heat Styling:

Hair styling is essential when you step out. You need to look good at all times in today's world. But it is necessary that you submit your hair to as less of heat treatment as you can! The heat tends to dry the shaft out making it dry and frizzy which over a period causes the hair to turn brittle. The ultimate result will be hair fall.

13. Avoid Hot Water For Hair Rinse:

Do not wash hair with hot water because excess heat is really bad for your hair. Always use cold water or water at room temperature. Dry and frizzy hair when you walk out of the shower is the indication that the water was too hot for your hair.

14. Healthy and Nutritious Diet:

All said and done, jut these simple precautions are not going to help. It will always hold true that only when you are healthy inside will your hair be healthy too. Your hair is made up of proteins and is alive at the roots. And like any other living it also requires nutrients to remain healthy and grow. There are a few things that you can add to your diet to ensure that you intake sufficient quantities of these nutrients.

First and foremost will be proteins of course. They are the building blocks of the hair shaft after all.

The next in the list will be vitamins. The vitamins that are essential for the hair are Vitamin A, B complex, C, and E. Each of these performs a significant role. Vitamin B complex is most popularly known for its importance in the hair growth and hair fall control. Vitamin C prevents premature graying.

Last but not the least, Iron. Deficiency of iron can lead to severe hair fall, which is why women suffering from anemia exhibit a great amount of hair fall.

15. Exercise:

Daily exercising also promotes hair growth. You must be wondering how? Exercise helps in improving metabolism. This allows better absorption of nutrients in your body. Exercise also helps to reduce stress. It releases endorphins or happy hormones which directly help in hair growth. When you are healthy and happy it shows on your skin and hair. So stay cheerful to have healthy glowing hair!

16. Reduce Your Caffeine Intake:

If you already have dry hair, then rethink your coffee habit and evaluate your caffeine consumption. Caffeine further depletes the body of its natural resources of nutrients. And the nutrients required for hair are not spared either! So cut back on the coffee and move on to something healthier and that which promotes good health.

17. Stay Hydrated:

Drink a lot of water and stay hydrated.

18. Use Herbal Products:

Keep the scalp clean and as far as possible away from chemicals. Use a herbal or Ayurvedic shampoo that is mild.

19. Regular Trim:

Trim your hair regularly to avoid the troubles of split ends. Keep your hair clean, use a thin comb to clear nits and head lice.

20. Avoid Residue Build-up:

Have a manageable hairstyle that helps to add volume to your hair. If you are using mousse or serum to add volume, make sure you rinse it off well during washing your hair with a shampoo. These residue stick to the hair follicles and create a breeding ground for dandruff and head lice.

A Word of Caution:

When you are using hair fall remedies at home it is necessary to keep a few tips in mind. Here they are:

Check to make sure that you aren't allergic to any of the ingredients mentioned in the hair products. Even though herbal products cause fewer reactions than chemicals, some people are known to have allergies to a few specific ingredients. Read labels of hair products carefully.

Always follow the instructions given in the product label carefully. If you don't follow the instructions carefully it will lead to hair fall again. It will do more harm than good.

While you follow these basic daily and weekly suggestions to reduce hair fall, you need to supplement it with some products that you can use everyday or twice during the week. Shampoos are the best example for such products. Supplementing these treatments with a good hair fall defense shampoo can be really useful.

Recommended Hair Products:

Here are a few good hair fall defense shampoo's you can try.

The Himalaya anti-hair fall shampoo

L'Oreal Paris new fall repair 3X Anti hair fall shampoo

Tresemme hair fall defense shampoo.

There are many more and make sure you try out a few and pick the one most suited to your hair. Remember your hair is precious and you need to pick what works the best for you!

Hair is the barometer of your health. Lead a healthy lifestyle if you want enviable tresses. You can flaunt any hair style with thick hair, so your aim should be to increase the volume of your hair naturally without using any hair serums. Now that you know the causes that trigger hair fall and methods to prevent it, you can take care of your hair even better. So no more embarrassing bald patches to hide! Let your hair shine with health.

Follow any of these simple home remedies and tips for hair loss / fall and get lustrous shining hair with regular practice.

60 Home Remedies to stop hair loss start hair regrowth Know everything about Hair loss and Hair regrowth

Home Remedies for Hair Loss baldness hair re growth Home Remedies to stop hair fall and increase hair growth

Hair loss is known as Khalitya Paalitya in Ayurveda. According to Ayurveda, People who have excess Pitta in their body are likely to lose their hair early in life, or have prematurely thin or gray hair.

Excess Pitta in the sebaceous gland, at the root of the hair, or folliculitis can lead to hair loss.

Human hair naturally grows in three phases:

1.

Anagen - Anagen is the active or growing phase.

2.

Catagen - Catagen is a short phase of the natural hair cycle during which hairs begin to break down.

3.

Telogen - Telogen is the resting phase. The hairs that are shed daily are often in the resting or late phase in the hair cycle.

Normally, about 10% of the scalp hairs are in the resting or telogen phase at any time. These hairs are not growing and are getting prepared for cyclic shedding.

The human scalp has around 1, 00,000 – 1, 50,000 hair follicles.

Each follicle grows a hair continuously up to age 8.

The average scalp has up to 150,000 hairs.

Each follicle produces a single hair that grows at a rate of half an inch per month.

After growing for two to six years, hair rests awhile before falling out.

It is soon replaced with a new hair, and the cycle begins again.

At any given time, 85% of hair is growing, and the remainder is resting.

Most people lose anywhere from 50 to 100 strands of hair each day, according to the American Academy of Dermatology

Hair loss is common in Women too.

Like men, females also face hair loss problem.

What is PH balance shampoo?

In advertisements popular shampoo brands use the term PH balanced shampoo so what is the meaning of pH balanced shampoo?

pH is a scale from 0 to 14, which measures the acidity or alkalinity of a solution.

Solutions with a pH less than 7 are acidic,

pH more than 7 are alkaline.

Solutions with a pH of 7 are considered neutral.

The natural pH of hair is around 5.5.

At this pH, the hair is the strongest

If a solution, which is either acidic or alkaline, is applied to hair, it will become weaker. Any chemical with a pH of more than 10, or less than 0 will severely damage hair.

Thus, balance of pH is very important in shampoo.

Everyone who is suffering from hair loss or facing baldness knows in his heart he got the problem and problem is visible to everyone.

For us important is home remedies, which will help to stop hair loss, stop growing baldness, or keep in control the hair loss and bald ness.

What is dandruff?

In short, it is a condition where the skin cells on the scalp go into over drive and are produced in excess, which gives rise to irritation and itching.

Dandruff is a condition where the skin cells on the scalp are produced in excess.

One can get dandruff on parts of your body other than your scalp, like your forehead, eyebrows, eyelashes, or ears.

Dandruff does not directly cause hair loss,

but scratching scalp a lot could cause hair loss.

Following are the few reasons of hair loss and baldness

1)

Hereditary or Hair loss that is genetic is known as androgenetic alopecia

2)

old age

3)

Protein deficiency

4)

Vitamin deficiency e.g. Deficiency of vitamin B12

5)

Anemia

6)

Hormonal imbalance

7)

Iron deficiency occasionally produces hair loss

8)

Tensions or Stress can cause hair loss

9)

Unhealthy Scalp - Skin conditions that lead to hair loss include seborrheic dermatitis (dandruff), psoriasis, and fungal infections such as ringworm.

10)

Thyroid abnormalities

11)

High doses of Vitamin A, blood pressure medications, Gout medications can also cause hair loss

Following are the home remedies, which will help to stop hair loss, start hair re growth, stop growing baldness, and increasing hair fall and hair loss.

For every person the reason for hair loss is different so one should try all the home remedies and keep watch on allergies when you will try home remedies.

2)

Hair loss reason – Hereditary – Reduce the hair loss by applying minoxidil (Rogaine) to the scalp twice a day. Women should not use minoxidil if they are pregnant or nursing. Men may be treated with finasteride (Propecia), an oral medication.

3)

Avoid Pitta-aggravating foods like spicy, and oily foods,

4)

Avoid or reduce consumption of tea and coffee.

5)

Avoid refined foods

6)

Avoid refined sugar

7)

Avoid junk food

8)

Avoid alcoholic drink

9)

Avoid carbonated drinks

10)

Start eating green leafy vegetables

11)

Start drinking vegetable juices prepared from lettuce, carrot, capsicum, and alfalfa.

12)

Mix Indian gooseberry (amla) and sesame seeds in equal amounts. Take 1 teaspoon twice a day with water.

13)

Heat 500 milliliters of coconut oil in a pan, and add 8 amla cut into pieces. Heat until the amla turn dark brown or black. Use the oil for a hair massage 2-3 times a week.

14)

Take 2 cup of curry leaves and grind them with 2 cup of buttermilk. Apply this to the hair for 1 hour, and then wash the hair

15)

boil some henna leaves in mustard oil. After cooling and straining this preparation, mix it in a coconut oil and start using this oil.

16)

wash the hair with a paste made from Neem leaves helps stop hair loss.

17)

washing the hair with apple cider vinegar reduces hair fall.

18)

Applying Curd to hair helps reduce dandruff.

19)

Do not brush the hair when it is wet. Let them dry.

20)

Start washing hairs with Aritha and Shikakai Powder. It does not have any chemicals or any other side effects. Aritha and Shikakai powder is available at any kirana store or general store.

21)

Do not use too hot water for hairs and scalp. It can damage the roots and may increase dandruff.

22)

Avoid using appliances that overheat your hair. Set your hair dryer on cool and low settings

23)

To stop hair fall, massage your scalp with fingers gently

24)

Always wear a cap with brim or a scarf to protect from sunlight

25)

always use a swimming cap or at least shampoo your hair after swimming.

26)

Apply coconut milk all over the scalp and massaging gently into the hair

27)

Apply juice of green coriander leaves on the head

28)

Apply Amla Oil, start using Amla Oil = to prepare amla oil, put some dry pieces of amla in coconut oil and bring to a boil and oil is ready for use.

29)

Brahmi and Bhringraj oil massage reduces or stops hair loss.

30)

Boil fresh neem leaves in water for an hour. Strain the water and let it cool. Wash hair with this neem leaves water.

31)

Boil curry leaves with coconut oil until leaves turn black. Strain the oil, and store in a bottle and use this oil for massage daily.

32)

Take 1-cup amla juice and 1-cup lemon juice mix it and apply it to hair, scalp and then wash the hairs.

33)

Hair loss – reason iron deficiency - start eating spinach every day or start iron pills with the advice of doctor. Eat iron-rich foods such as beef, pork, fish, leafy greens, fortified cereals, and beans

34)

Zinc also helps stop hair loss so start eating wholegrain flour

35)

Eat food, which contains vitamin B, Vitamin C, Vitamin E.

36)

Copper stops hair loss – Start eating nuts cashews and peanuts, seeds, whole milk and beans

37)

Start eating almonds

38)

Apply almond oil on scalp and massage

39)

Massage warm castor oil mixed with almond oil into your scalp gently. Wrap a hot towel around your scalp so it gets absorbed into the hair. Do this 2 or 3 times a week

40)

Grind fenugreek seeds in water and apply on your scalp. Wash off after 30 minutes or 1 hour. Do it for 1 month and helps you do it every day until full satisfaction.

41)

Start eating Amla or drinking Amla Juice.

42)

Using a 5% tea tree oil shampoo may reduce dandruff and that itchy feeling.

43)

Dandruff – Massage the Scalp with pure coconut oil or apply lemon juice to scalp before washing hair.

44)

Ketoconazole fights dandruff-causing fungus.

45)

Dandruff - Salicylic acid gets rid of flaky skin but can be drying.

46)

Dandruff - Selenium sulfide slows the buildup of dead skin cells and fights fungi.

47)

Dandruff - Tar slows dead skin cell buildup, but may discolor blonde, gray, or color-treated hair.

48)

Aloe. Using aloe on the scalp may help reduce itchiness and scaliness.

49)

Zinc pyrithione attacks the fungi that may cause dandruff.

50)

Lemongrass shampoo. Washing with a 2%, lemongrass shampoo may help fight fungus that causes dandruff.

51)

Best foods for hairs =Salmon, walnuts, Oysters, egg, milk, sweet potato, spinach, lentils, yogurt , blueberries, Kiwis, tomatoes, strawberries, lemon, amla

52)

Coconut oil, rosemary oil, brahmi and bhringraj oil, vitamin E oil all these oils are best for hair scalp massage always massage gently.

53)

Start drinking Aloe Vera juice.

54)

Applying Aloe Vera extract to your scalp can greatly reduce the hair fall and help regrowth of the hair.

55)

Garlic and onion – help stop hair fall and regrowth Star using herbal oils which contain garlic or onion extract.

56)

To slow down hair loss you can try These medications like Minoxidil, Propecia, and Avodart and prostaglandin analogs

57)

Try multivitamin Tablets, which contain zinc, vitamin B, folate, iron, and calcium, Vitamin D, Vitamin C or try combination of vitamin pills.

58)

White hair - Take a tablespoon of amla and almond oil. Mix few drops of limejuice to it and apply on your scalp.

59)

White hair - apply mixture of limejuice, amla juice, and almond oil. To make the mixture take 4 tablespoon of almond oil, 1 tablespoon of amla and lemon juice. Gently massage on scalp and leave for 1 hour.

60)

Rubbing left and right hand's fingernails with each other is a powerful technique for curing hair fall and increasing hair growth. 4 fingernails of right hand and left hand rub them each other. Thumb fingernails of left and right hand are not rubbed on each other. Fold both your palms inwards and place the fingernails of both hands against each other. Then with regular swift motions, rub them against each other. It is free of cost and you can do it any time anywhere while watching TV or listening music, do it daily 5 to 20 minutes everyday twice.

Don't rub your thumbnails because it will accelerate the growth of beard, moustache or facial hairs.

Avoid it during Pregnancy

www.ingramcontent.com/pod-product-compliance
Lightning Source LLC
Chambersburg PA
CBHW071154280526
45787CB00003B/1506